Your Quest for a Spiritual Life

Based on Patanjali's Sutras

For Everyone on Their Spiritual
Journey Seeking Guidance

First published by O Books, 2010
O Books is an imprint of John Hunt Publishing Ltd., The Bothy, Deershot Lodge, Park Lane, Ropley,
Hants, SO24 0BE, UK
office1@o-books.net
www.o-books.net

Distribution in:

UK and Europe
Orca Book Services
orders@orcabookservices.co.uk
Tel: 01202 665432 Fax: 01202 666219
Int. code (44)

USA and Canada
NBN
custserv@nbnbooks.com
Tel: 1 800 462 6420 Fax: 1 800 338 4550

Australia and New Zealand
Brumby Books
sales@brumbybooks.com.au
Tel: 61 3 9761 5535 Fax: 61 3 9761 7095

Far East (offices in Singapore, Thailand,
Hong Kong, Taiwan)
Pansing Distribution Pte Ltd
kemal@pansing.com
Tel: 65 6319 9939 Fax: 65 6462 5761

South Africa
Stephan Phillips (pty) Ltd
Email: orders@stephanphillips.com
Tel: 27 21 4489839 Telefax: 27 21 4479879

Text copyright Michelle Corrigan 2009

Design: Stuart Davies

ISBN: 978 1 84694 295 2

A CIP catalogue record for this book is available
from the British Library.

Printed by Digital Book Print

O Books operates a distinctive and ethical publishing philosophy in
all areas of its business, from its global network of authors to
production and worldwide distribution.

Your Quest
for a Spiritual Life

Based on Patanjali's Sutras

For Everyone on Their Spiritual
Journey Seeking Guidance

Michelle Corrigan

BOOKS

Winchester, UK
Washington, USA

CONTENTS

Notes on the Author

My Yoga journey began many moons ago in 1994 whilst on a two-year expatriate spell in Bangkok. I often visited the beautiful Thai Buddhist temples and went on a Meditation retreat run by Buddhist Monks which was in the form of Vipassana Meditation - insight meditation focusing on the breath and repeating mantras (sacred sounds) on the rise and fall of the abdomen. Whilst in Bangkok, I also studied Thai massage - a wonderful body treatment of pressing the energy lines with the thumbs and palms of the hands.

I then trained as an Aromatherapist in Dorking, England; this is a lovely body massage using bespoke aromatherapy oils, tracing meridians making this a holistic treatment.

Whilst living in Devon I trained as a Reiki Practitioner which introduced me to the esoteric body system. I also joined a meditation group which helped me with expanding the technique of visualisation and opened up my spiritual awareness.

In 2002, I moved to Surrey with my family and set up my own meditation and healing groups and in 2004 I started my training with the British Wheel of Yoga as a Yoga Teacher.

I realised that my path is to do deep soul work and seek liberation so I have also spent time doing self-study and healing. I have spent some years looking at the self, discovering who I am, my purpose for being here and healing the soul. I have found Shamanic Healing really effective - Journeying and Soul Retrieval.

Shamanism is about being connected to the earth and nature, as well as being connected to the Great Divine. Many people believe that Shamanism is only connected to the Native American Energies, however it is about the old ways of living, honouring the Earth, the food that it provides and honouring the Sun and The Moon. As it states in the sutras - we all have the Sun (Male) and Moon (Female) energies within us, this also relates to the Yin and Yang theory from the Far East. These old theories have never really been lost but have been suppressed over the years. These philosophies are very similar at their core but the teachings vary. However to me they all lead to the same common wholeness. What is this wholeness? There are many answers to this question but for me it is union of the mind, body and spirit, being in touch with the self, knowing who you are, being at peace and in harmony, being liberated from suffering. When you are in harmony and at peace with the self, you have an abundance of energy, energy which can be sent out into the universe to help in the healing of the planet.

When on your Yoga mat practicing the postures, breathing techniques and meditating, enjoying the peace, finding balance, experiencing Samadhi, the balance doesn't stop there. When you roll up your mat, you take with you this peace of mind and use it in your every day life. Be mindful, even when doing tasks such as washing up, try not to let the mind race around taking you into the past, thinking about the future, be in the moment, the present, the now.

My Sanskrit name given to me by my great Yoga tutor - Swami Satchidananda Mataji, is "Mokshapriya" which means "She for who liberation is dear". In numerology, I am a number 5 which means I am here to do soul work and work as a Master Healer and Spiritual Teacher, to pass on the higher truth.

Introduction

We are constantly seeking outside of ourselves for answers, for happiness, joy and fulfillment, when everything we need is inside of ourselves, it is just a matter of knowing how to access this wisdom.

As a spiritual seeker, find the essence of who you are, connect to your soul, find peace and balance and be in this beautiful place.

Then your beautiful energy can be sent out to others and the Universe.

This is my interpretation of the Yoga Sutras. There are a few different translations of Patanjali's Yoga Sutras (written in Sanskrit at least two thousand years ago) but I felt it necessary to do my own version which I hope is easy for you to understand and connect with. The reason for this, is because I feel that the sutras are accessible to all, not just those who do Yoga.

I strongly felt a need to use these threads of wisdom in a way that we can connect to in the West. We can integrate what we learn from these Eastern philosophies into our lives that we lead.

This version of the sutras is aimed at anyone on their spiritual paths who need guidance and for those who practice Yoga.

The Yoga Sutras are for all cultures, races, religions and backgrounds. Yoga is not just about the physical which is the postures (asana), it is about union of the mind, body and spirit. By studying the sutras, a deeper understanding of this triad will evolve within you. A lot of people come into Yoga through the posture work and think it is just a physical form of exercise however it works on a much deeper level if you find the right teacher who is practicing with the right intent and who has studied the sutras themselves, then they may help you on your path. Once you start looking into the self; the mind, the spirit and the body, then you are beginning to walk your spiritual path.

I have read several different versions of these sutras, some of which I found quite difficult to understand and I hope that my version will help you, as a householder in these modern times (rather than a Yogi living in a cave for years), to understand the self more.

In the old times, students would have been able to devote their whole lives to their spiritual practice by going off into caves or walking to sacred places. This is not practical today as we have families, jobs - our earthly lives to lead.

One thing that all human beings have in common is that we are all connected to the Great Divine. It doesn't matter what religion or philosophy you follow; we all have the ability to walk out of the darkness and into the light. The soul can then head back home to a place that is home for us all.

These threads of wisdom will remind you to look within for answers.

Remember, we are all one consciousness, there is no separation.

Chapter 1

Samadhi Pada - Concentration

The Yoga Sutras are in four chapters. The first chapter is Samadhi Pada which examines the art of concentration, and teaches how to focus and meditate. The mind is very hard to train and control and this chapter discusses the mind; how busy it is and the distractions it faces. How our mind can be both our friend and our enemy, how it can be heavy sending out negative thoughts and sometimes even depressive thoughts. How the mind can be energetic with thoughts racing around in our heads or in the light state - where the mind can be calm and serene.

The goal is Samadhi. This state of consciousness is a state that we experience in meditation - a blissful, peaceful, enlightened state. To reach that goal, we must practice regularly and work on healing the self. The sutras also mention that although Samadhi is the goal, once reached, the work is not all done. Don't take a step back and think that is it, the spiritual path carries on and we never stop learning. Once Samadhi has been attained the higher truth can be revealed.

These wisdoms remind us to have awareness, be in the present.

Enjoy your quest. Don't just see the end - the goal, the journey is part of the wholeness.

1.1

Start doing Yoga from where you are now. Not from where you were yesterday, not tomorrow, not next week. Start from the present. Here begins the teachings of Yoga with the right intent at the right time - **now.** If you seek a class or teacher (which is advisable), find a teacher who you feel comfortable with, that creates the right energy in the room, that is in touch with the students. Use your discernment.

1.2

Yoga is stillness of the mind - to have focus, and not allow the chitter chatter to distract. When the mind is still, everything is still.

Citta means mind which means consciousness that connects the mind to the soul. Citta is part of three components - mind (manas), intelligence (buddhi) and ego (ahamkara) which are combined together as a whole.

Yoga gives you peace of mind and liberates you from the activity of the mind. Yoga will bring you calmness and balance. Once your mind is at peace, then the benefits will manifest in the physical body bringing harmony and health.

1.3

When the mind is silent and at peace, the true self is revealed. The connection to the soul can be made. It is like a pool of still water, with no ripples or waves, the water becomes crystal clear.

1.4

At other times, when not in this Yogic state, the mind is busy and will wander.

In time you will come to understand your truths and your mind will not try and distract you away from your truths, for clarity will replace confusion.

1.5

The mind can fluctuate and this creates variations in your thoughts. Thoughts can be painful (klista) i.e.: negative, horrid, dark, self-sabotaging, or thoughts can be non-painful (aklistah), more positive, bright, kind, etc.

1.6

The five classes of movements of the mind are: right knowledge, wrong knowledge, imagination, sleep and memory.

These five categories of movement of the mind are:

- Right knowledge - a proven theory which has been reliably sourced.
- Wrong knowledge - assumptions and presumptions.
- Imagination - fanciful or imaginary knowledge which could include delusion.
- Sleep - knowledge based on sleep and dreams.
- Memory - recollection of thoughts from the past.

1.7

Right knowledge is gained from words and actions of Spiritual Teachers - by joining a Yoga Class, going to Meditation Groups, finding a suitable person who you believe is coming from the right place (is this knowledge *their* own interpretation, or is it true?) Your teacher should be someone who you feel comfortable with, they should be approachable and when they teach they should be sharing their knowledge with you and not preaching. You should feel warmth in their presence. Use discernment when choosing your spiritual teacher and follow your intuition.

After being with your Teacher, you should feel empowered.

Right knowledge is based on spiritual intelligence, intuition, actual testimony from sacred texts and scriptures or direct from The Masters in Spirit through channelling. Channelling philosophy can be done by those who have mastered the gift in linking to The Great Masters in Spirit.

1.8

Wrong knowledge is caused by error, misconception, or by mistaking one thing for another i.e.: you see a bird out the corner of your eye and believe it to be an eagle. You look closer and find that in fact it is a pheasant. From a glimpse you made an assumption rather than being patient and sure and seeing it for what it is. Wrong understanding and wrong knowledge will generate blocks on your spiritual path. Your perception will be clouded and your feelings will be unsettled.

1.9

When words are spoken, we can often jump to conclusions. Our imagination takes over, leading us to conclusions which may have no substance and this a sign of weakness of the mind.

When in the presence of your Teacher, allow words of wisdom to sink in. Try and digest wise words and allow them to be, without analysing everything and making your own assumptions. Let the true depth of these words come through and then, the truth can become clear rather than truths without substance. When a Master speaks, listen, do not try and think about a reply or analyze the words, or judge, just listen and absorb.

1.10

Nidra or Lucid Dreaming is a state of consciousness where there is an absence of thought-waves, but there is still a trace of consciousness. When meditating, you should not fall asleep, 'sleep is sleep' and 'meditation is meditation'. (Saying by Theravada Buddhist Monk in Thailand).

Sleep is where the state of consciousness is in a place where everyday thoughts do not clutter the mind but where dreams take place. Not all dreams are prophetic but some are and carry powerful messages.

1.11

Memory is a recollection of past experiences and words.

These experiences continue to live within you and these can be both positive and negative. Our conditioning from the past is imprinted in our memory and that is why we find it difficult to break old habits. Past experiences may not be forgotten in the mind but they can be healed from the soul. Cellular memory is where emotions are stored in the cells of the body, for instance in the muscles and it is believed that by stretching the muscles through postures, that releases take place.

1.12

To reach the state of Yoga, you should practice regularly. Learn non-attachment, not in the sense of detaching yourself from your family, your work or any of your earthly energies but in the sense of studying your own attachments imprinted in your mind. By practising Yoga - Asana, Pranayama, Meditation and studying the texts, you will detach yourself from the Sanskaras -imprints left on the sub-conscious mind by experience.

1.13

Regular effort and practice will result in a more balanced mind. Peace will be in the mind, will be felt in the heart, the body will be more in harmony and the soul will be obtainable.

1.14

Devote yourself to your regular Yoga practice and you will grow. The results will not happen immediately but will take continuous effort and dedication. Wisdom will shine through you and around you. At times you will need a Master and often when the time is right they will appear in your life. At other times you will need to ground your teachings and process your healing, sometimes you should be the Hermit - allow the trans-formation to take place, find space alone and let the wisdom shine through.

1.15

Renunciation is the practice of letting go of your desires and passions. Letting go of your attachments is liberation of desires. This will result in you being in a more peaceful space, the mind not hankering after desires but being content. These desires could be in the form of material possessions, foods that you crave but do not really need such as another piece of chocolate, wanting to move house if there is nothing wrong with where you are, buying a new television just because a new model has come in when there is nothing wrong with the one you have. The desires could be coming from the ego and also could be in the form of wanting the siddhis - the psychic powers. These desires will distract you from your true spiritual path as they are not the goal and these powers alone will not give you liberation.
Let your deep inner knowing lead you and not your ego.

1.16

Non-attachment is being free, being your true self with no distractions. According to Yoga philosophy, the whole of nature consists of three qualities known as The Gunas - Tamas - heavy, inertia, Rajas - energetic, lively, vibrancy and Sattvic - light, luminosity, serenity. We can apply these three qualities to our mind (heavy, lively, calm), to our physical body (inertia, energetic, balanced), to the animal kingdom, to the plant kingdom, food etc.
Letting go comes with self-development by understanding these qualities of nature within the self.
An example would be, what makes your body and mind feel heavy, let's take a certain food that you know makes you feel heavy, this would usually be **too much** red meat, dairy, alcohol,

caffeine or sugar. When you consume this tamasic food, then the body will be in a tamasic state - lethargic. When you eat rajasic food, then the body will be all over the place - fidgety. So when you eat sattvic food, the body and mind will feel lighter. When you are in tune with the self, then the soul can be seen and you will then be working at a deeper level, free from attachments. Then you will be in a more balanced space.

1.17

A state of Samadhi can then be reached. Samadhi is a state of full concentration, the mind is totally focused. There are different levels of Samadhi - one level is where there is still awareness of your body even though you are deeply focused. Another level is where you have no awareness of being in your body; you have raised your consciousness out of the body.

The results are knowledge and wisdom. Realization of the gifts of reasoning, or the ability to analyze - when it is appropriate, the gift of discrimination or discernment - using your better judgment on situations and even people - really seeing what is there, the gift of bliss (ananda) and the gift of awareness of the truth and your own true self.

See it as like a cloud being lifted away; then seeing clear blue sky.

1.18

The memories of our life do not leave us altogether but will be there to help us to continue through life rather than distract us in our practice. This state of Samadhi is where the mind is still, it is not disturbing us but is in a pure peaceful state. Concentration can be obtained during Asana, Pranayama and Meditation. Samadhi seems to be a place that we can all reach, feel this blissful state and then when we are going about our daily duties and earthly experiences harmony and balance can be felt. The mind will be more focused and you will be able to live in the moment.

1.19

When practising meditation, you should feel connected to Mother Earth (nature, the ground) first, only then should you attempt to open the upper chakras and connect to Spirit. It is very tempting to try to connect to Angels, Spirit Guides, Ascended Masters before you are ready (a good teacher will know and understand) but first your energies must be grounded.

1.20

Trust what you believe to be your truth using your own experiences which you have learnt from the real knowledge of The Teachers and Wise Sages.

Once you have attained a certain level in Samadhi, it will take your own self-discipline and trust to keep going and not think that you have learnt it all as we never stop learning. It is vital to keep focused, using your experiences with The Masters and to know for yourself what is real knowledge.

1.21

The goal is within reach to those who practice regularly, are focused and are sincere with their intent. There will be obstacles on your path and these will be challenges for you to overcome, to make you grow so your soul can evolve - for your wisdom to come through.

1.22

The more energy you put in to your practice, the more you will get out of it. Of course your own circumstances will dictate what time and energy you have but it is important to allow yourself this space regularly without any disturbances. Again self-discipline is needed and the factor of how hungry are you to reach these goals, how important is it for you in your life to be in

Samadhi? What are your priorities? What effort are your prepared to put into your yoga practice? Perhaps you think once a week attending a class is enough, perhaps you practice every day with full effort and energy.

1.23

Patanjali refers to Isvara in this sutra, which in Yoga philosophy is translated as 'God', 'Lord', 'Universal Soul'.

(Myself I tend to use the phrase 'The Great Divine'. You may have your own words for this energy which is greater than the self. Other cultures have their own word(s) for their God or icon. It is my belief that we as humans have individual souls and in another dimension is "The Great Divine" - the Universal Soul. I believe that we have been led to believe that we are separate but in fact we are one great consciousness and through the practice of Yoga and connecting to the soul, clearing our chakras, we become closer to this universal consciousness).

There comes a time in your practice where you can feel this great energy around you and you start to really feel connected and this sutra is about surrendering, letting go and trusting.

1.24

'Who is God'?

Meditate on this question, find your own truths; Who do you pray to? What do you feel connected to?

(We should remember that the sutras are based upon Hindu and Buddhist philosophy and perhaps you could think about the idea of God being a separate energy or God being One Energy with the self. What feels right to you?)

1.25

This Great Spirit Energy (The Great Divine, God) is omnipresent (all-present), omniscient (knowing all), omnipotent (all-powerful).

1.26

In spirit, there is no time. There is only timelessness.

1.27

If you chant "OM" you will connect to this Great Energy.

1.28

Om is a mantra, a sacred sound and by repeating this either in your head or out loud, with feeling, the energy of this sound will be heard by The Great Divine. The sound will resonate and the vibration will connect.

1.29

Chanting OM will help with focus, the mind will become clearer. This practice will help to remove obstacles and clear the energy centre at the throat.

1.30

What are the obstacles?

Disease, inertia, doubt, carelessness, sluggishness, lack of discipline, distorted views, being ungrounded and lack of perseverance.

If we do not pay attention to these obstacles, then you cannot reach the state of Yoga.

1.31

Dukha - sorrow and pain

Are you becoming aware of any of these obstacles and what can you do about them? Having awareness means you are on the road to healing. This sutra talks about the sorrow and pain that are part of the obstacles, the unsteadiness of the body, the mental negativity, irregular breathing which further distract you.

As you focus on your breath, observe your inhale, as you exhale, blow away any negative emotions, grief or fears. Do not rush the breathing techniques, Pranayama is an equally important part of your Yoga practice.

Look after your physical body for it is your vehicle to take you through life. Recognise when you are feeling heavy - study the gunas. Trust instead of doubting. Do not be careless when you practice Yoga - be mindful and present. Sluggishness can be either mental or physical - be more positive, stand upright and walk your path with your head high. Be disciplined with your practice - regularity is the key. When learning from The Masters, interpret into your own words without distorting the truth. Always work on being grounded, start your practice by being connected to the Earth, visualize a Oak tree with roots going deep into the ground. There will be times during your Yoga practice where you will feel you are not progressing, have patience, keep going.

You may experience shaking of the body during practice, do not worry, this is just the body responding to your powerful Yoga practice, energy is shifting. Slowly wind down from your practice for that day (see Sutra 2.46 on Asana).

1.32

Practice the various techniques of steadying the mind and find the one that suits you.

The basic technique for focusing the mind during asana would be to focus on your breath, work with the breath during the movement. For example with a forward bend, inhale raise the arms, exhale as you go into the forward bend, inhale come out of the posture with arms by ears, exhale lower the arms. Your mind should be on the breath, the movement and being aware of the physical body.

1.33

Dukha - sorrow and pain
Sukha - happiness and joy

In life we go through stages and experiences of both sorrow and pain, and happiness and joy. To know what happiness and joy is, we have to experience the sorrow and pain.

Be compassionate to yourself and others when in the suffering and pain experience.

Have positive people around you and allow yourself to feel love, happiness and joy.

Rejoice when in the company of your Spiritual Teacher. When in the company of an evolved Teacher, you should feel and see their peace, joy, balance and happiness.

Be aware that you may be attached to the feeling of happiness and joy and are not able to cope with the other emotions of sadness, anger, hatred and pain and your way of dealing with dukha is to suppress these emotions.

1.34

Use the breath as your object of focus.

Focus on extending the exhale.

Inhale, natural pause, exhale to the full extent of your breath, pause.

Use the full length of your breath, the full capacity of your lungs, do not rush.

1.35

Use the senses as your focus for meditation:

Breath in, pause, breath out, pause. Softly focus on a spot on the floor. Close the eyes. Focus on one sense at a time - hearing, smell, seeing, taste, touch. Firstly focus on the ears, listen. Focus on the nose, the sense of smell will grow stronger. Focus on the eyes, see. Focus on the mouth - taste. Focus on your skin, feel. Gently open your eyes.

1.36

Here, the concentration is on the heart.

Focus on your heart. Visualise a beautiful pink lotus flower with the petals open. Feel the love all around you. Allow this love into your heart with every inhale. Exhale any negative emotions you may be holding on to. Repeat, over and over.

Gently open the eyes.

We often give love out to others and omit receiving love ourselves.

1.37

Here use an iconic statue such as a statue of Buddha for your object of focus. It could also be a picture of your Master, a Divine being such as Sri Swami Sivananda, Paramahansa Yogananda, i.e.: an enlightened Sage who is free from desires and attachments and at peace.

There will be times when you can overcome your obstacles and challenges through meditation or there will be other times where you may need to turn to a wise sage to talk over your problems, a therapist. When we are confronted with problems, or issues arise, it is often helpful to seek counsel from someone qualified who can empathise with you, possibly someone who has experienced similar things. There are many different types of helpful therapy available today. It is not a weakness to need a therapist; it needs strength and courage. A good therapist will make you feel empowered.

1.38

In your sleep state, your mind cannot come in and intervene. Wisdom often comes through dreams. If you seek guidance on something then before you go to sleep, ask The Great Divine. If you wake in the night and your guidance comes in the form of a dream, it is advisable to write this down, as often, by the time morning comes, the dream is forgotten.

Sometimes it is useful to meditate on your dream also when you are in the waking state, to commune with The Great Divine for guidance.

1.39

Still the mind by meditating on an object. For this technique use the self as the object. Take your focus to different parts of the body. Feel the breath. Focus on the seven main energy centres up the spine (see sutra 3.27). Focus on the energy around you. Connect to The Great Energy around you.

1.40

The mind can be freed of all disturbances. You become one with your object of meditation.

1.41

If you meditate on a object such as a tree, feel you are at one with the tree. See the roots going deep into Mother Earth, feel how grounded that feels. Feel the strong steady trunk and feel your spine straight and having the strength to hold your body. See the leaves, be the leaves. See the branches reaching up to the sky and see yourself branching out to The Great Divine.

1.42

Your hidden wisdoms can shine through. Your mind cannot intervene with the real truth. The intelligence is freed from conditioning.

1.43

Your mind is at peace, it doesn't seek what is stored in your memory. The mind becomes pure and clear, just like a crystal.

1.44

The distractions are absent and the light becomes crystal clear. Your senses are quiet, there is just pure energy.

1.45

There is still an awareness of consciousness. There is still an element of being earthed.

1.46

The seeds of the past are still there, deeply planted. But for the moment you have reached a level of Samadhi.

1.47

You are experiencing a Sattvic state - mentally, physically and emotionally. You will be in touch with your soul, your true essence.

1.48

Your wisdom and truth will shine through. An awakening is taking place.

1.49

You will find your own words to describe this level of consciousness. You will discover your own experiences and self-realizations.

1.50

When you go about your daily life, you will feel lighter, more balanced. You will gain insights and you will walk further down your spiritual path.

1.51

Life is about cycles. You will have come one full circle and are now ready for more soul work. You have come so far and you have started to see but there is more work to do.

·

CHAPTER 2

Sadhana Pada - Practice and Discipline

Now you have an understanding of how the mind works and how it can distract you. This is the chapter on practices. We are told how to practice, through discipline, study and dedication to an ideal, i.e.: an energy greater than ourselves. We learn about our obstacles to growth and how we can overcome them. This chapter talks about Kriya Yoga - self-discipline is required for you to practice Yoga on a regular basis. You have to keep putting more energy in and like anything else, you will get more back.

Karma is mentioned in chapter II - how your past actions can affect you later on. How we are responsible for every action, deed and thought - for as we sow, so shall we reap.

The kleshas are brought to your awareness here - the obstacles to your spiritual path. How ignorance blocks our view.

Patanjali's eight limbs of Yoga are discussed which gives insight on your outlook to others as well as your attitude towards yourself. This explains the different steps of growth.

The third, fourth and fifth limbs of Ashtanga Yoga are explained - Asana (postures), Pranayama (breathing) and Pratyahara (going inwards) and how the breath work is really important to practice.

We learn in this chapter that the search is within the self. It is like discovering a golden key - to unlock the wisdom.

2.1

We start this chapter with Kriya Yoga. Now you have come this far with your practice, discipline will be needed for you to walk further down your spiritual path. You may have achieved a level of Samadhi, it doesn't mean to say you have reached enlightenment. Kriya Yoga is composed of three actions - "tapas" – self-discipline, "svadhyaya" - self-study, and "Isvara pranidhanani" - surrender to the Great Divine.

Tapas - a level of discipline is required for you to fit in your daily Yoga practice; asana, pranayama, meditation as well as studying texts. It is very easy to put off doing our practice or let other tasks have priority.

Svadhyaya - self-study - as well as studying the self, this also refers to studying sacred texts which will help you in understanding the self. When you start to understand the self and the soul's purpose, then you will start to connect to the soul.

There are many different ways and techniques of understanding the individual self. To start you could find out what elements you are composed of (from your birth signs - horoscope) either fire, earth, water or air. You could find out a bit about yourself by looking at numerology if that appeals to you. Find out what energy you are working with by summing up the total number of your birth date and then finding out what that number means. This is again useful in understanding yourself.

Also learn from those around you. Often your great teachers are members of your family. Look at those people who stir within you hatred, anger, irritation as well as love, compassion, empathy and kindness; are they mirroring these emotions to you?

Isvara pranidhanani - connecting to The Great Divine through meditation, prayer and Mantra. Find a technique that suits you. Try meditating on "OM".

You can meditate on OM by saying it in your head or by chanting it out loud. For example, take an inhale, then on the exhale say the word "OM out loud. Observe how this lengthens your exhale.

Practice the chant whilst doing your postures. For example, on a flanked forward bend (parsvottanasana) - inhale raise the arms, exhale chant OM as you forward bend, inhale and come out of the posture raising the arms, exhale lower the arms. Repeat several times on each side.

Another way would be to play a CD with the chanting of OM.

Draw the symbol in large print and use this as your object of concentration.

See which method works for you.

2.2

The practice of Yoga will take you on your path to Samadhi. Kriya Yoga will bring you mind-control, self-awareness and will connect you to The Great Divine.

2.3

The obstacles on your path are:

Avidya - spiritual ignorance

Asmita - ego

Raga - desire and attachment

Dvesa - hatred and anger

Abhinivesah - fear

These are known as the kleshas - the five afflictions.

Avidya is the root of the problem and is the basis of the other four.

2.4

Most people go through life unaware of their spiritual paths. Some might say they are "blissfully ignorant" as once you start self-study your own wounds will surface. Whilst these wounds are processed and transformation takes place through active awareness, it can be difficult at times. Unaware people may never find true peace and happiness.

Spiritual ignorance will only suppress these wounds.

2.5

This period of healing can bring pains (dukha) as the wounds heal.

This will be followed by joy and pleasure (sukha) as you feel like a heavy weight has been lifted from your shoulders.

2.6

Asmita is egoism - pride, the "I am".

The Soul is the seer - pure spirit consciousness. The buddhi is where the ego sits in the mind. The ego can be seen as an obstacle to your true self as it takes upon itself to try to connect to the soul as it sees itself as the seer. The true seer is the soul.

The mind is not the true self, Atma - the seer is the true self.

The ego is seen as a Male energy - Sun energy. Too little of this energy may result in low self-esteem and low confidence, and too much of this energy may result in an inflated opinion of the self; overly confident and selfish.

It takes much experience to understand when ego is leading you or whether it is your intuition - your deep voice of knowing. The ego tries very hard to control us but in fact the Sutras talk about renunciation of the ego - letting go, being in control rather than letting the ego lead.

2.7

Raga is attachment to a desire.

It is very easy to become attached to pleasure and happiness. You may think an object will satisfy your desire. It could do initially, but in time there will be consequences. For example, if you desire a new car when the car you already have is quite functional and reliable and fits your needs, and you go out and purchase this new car (pleasure) with a three year financial loan because you have not got the cash for it. You may then spend the next three years struggling (pain) to pay for the loan on a car that you didn't really need in the first place.

Another example is the desire for a piece of cake full of sugar and cream (pleasure). Deep down you know that the piece of cake won't be good for your troubled digestive system but you eat it anyway. Later on you suffer indigestion, the pain from satisfying a desire.

Raga is wanting something that perhaps you have previously experienced which brought you pleasure, but is not necessarily something you actually need.

When your mind is full of desires, then you are practicing attachment. The Sutras often mention renunciation of attachments.

2.8

Dvesah - is aversion, hatred, abhorrence.

The mind can become attached to those things which bring us sorrow and pain - dukha - such as unfulfilled desires, hatred to others or the self, dwelling on wounds. This will lead to being self-absorbed, being the victim and will block your spiritual growth.

Once in this painful state it is like a spiral going down and down, it is then a huge challenge to come up again.

2.9

Abinivesa is fear. For example fear of death.

Fears are blocks to our paths.

Most people have a fear of dying. Death of the physical body is not death of the soul - it is going home to the spirit world. Upon death, as the very last exhale is taken, the soul will leave the physical body and pass over into the world of spirit - The Great Divine Consciousness.

When in a true Yogic state it is possible to feel the spirit within connecting to the Great Spirit around, then all fears will be lost.

2.10

These afflictions are subtle and are not obvious unless self-study is practiced.

2.11

Meditation and reflection will help to heal the kleshas (afflictions).

Contemplation and reflection is needed and can be achieved through prayer, meditation or discussion with a Wise Sage or Therapist/Healer. Sometimes others can see what you cannot see for yourself.

2.12

By working on the soul healing wounds from this life and attachments to past lives, the spirit can be free.

You will be here in this life with certain lessons and challenges. Understand what you are here to do. (Numerology is a great help for this).

2.13

Karma

Before you incarnated into this life, your soul will have chosen what circumstances to be born into; your family, surroundings, environment. Through your ancestors, your bloodline will bring you gifts and freedoms and also limitations and burdens. This is seen as family karma. This will give you the necessary learning for your soul to evolve.

You will be born with individual karma, actions from past lives that has generated karma that could be good or bad or a mixture of both.

You can study your family karma by observing your family patterns, behaviours; the gifts and freedoms your parents give you as well as burdens and limitations . So much can be discovered.

Your imprints from this life is known as samskaras and imprints from past lives are known as vasanas. These imprints are the seeds you have sewn; your past actions. You may not be aware of these past actions but they are imprinted in your sub-conscious. If you chose to work on this, then certain Therapists may help but be aware that it is the soul seeking this, not the ego. Going into past lives can be very painful, can be damaging to the mind if the environment is not right or adequate support is not available. It is thought by some that regressing into past lives can help with healing and shifting wounds and patterns that you carry in this life. Often when working at a deep level images of past lives can appear anyway, if this happens attach-ments should not be made.

2.14

Past actions bear fruit and depending on what the action was, good or bad, will decide whether the fruit bears pleasure or pain.

2.15

Once you have recognized bad actions, thoughts, then already the Karma is starting to release. Being aware is the key. Don't think that because you made a mistake in the past, you are going to pay for it by pain now. Recognize your mistake and genuinely learn from the lesson.

Even negative thought waves are sent out to the Universe so if you think something harsh about someone, try and correct yourself and send out positive thoughts.

Energy follows thought.

2.16

Do not hold on to past pain. Do not hold on to guilt; it is a waste of energy.

Observe the kleshas (afflictions) in sutra 2.3 and see how they effect you so you can avoid any pain that has not yet befallen. See it as untying chains around you - be free.

The pain which has not yet come may be avoided.

2.17

Ground your issues, problems, past actions. A good way of grounding issues would be to go out in nature, ask Mother Earth to take your sorrows and pains, or to sit on pebbles or rocks on a beach, or visit sacred stone circles such as Avebury or Stonehenge in the UK. All countries have sacred places.

Try seeking out an old tree such as Oak or Yew, look at the tree and see the strong trunk with the roots spreading out into Mother Earth. See these roots as taking your wounds and issues out of your head, out of your body, into the ground. Lift your arms in the air like the branches in the tree - be free.

Do not hang on to your baggage - let go.

Do not beat yourself up. Move on.

2.18

How you regard things and how you perceive them will have an effect on the energy you are putting out to the Universe. If your thoughts are negative, then you will send out negative energy to the Universe. If your thoughts are full of love, peace and joy, then this beautiful energy will be sent out to the Universe.

Sometimes our perception on reality brings pain, anger, sorrow and conflict. However it is only our perception which may differ from the reality - like a double edged sword. Your perception will dictate whether the mind will be positive or negative and sometimes there is a need to cut through the illusions that our mind creates. Awareness is half the battle.

2.19

Your state of mind will dictate how you are feeling, how you are emotionally and how you are feeling physically.

2.20

The quality of perception depends on the state of the mind.

2.21

All that is in your life - people, lessons, challenges, experiences is for the soul to grow and evolve.

2.22

The seer starts to see; you become more in touch with your soul. You become at one with The Universe.

2.23

You get to know your own true self.

2.24

Lack of awareness and spiritual knowledge (avidya) has to be overcome or you will stay stagnant.

2.25

Once this ignorance has been recognized, awareness is present and liberation is found. This is kaivalya.

2.26

Overcome confusion, then you have clarity. This requires constant effort and energy.

Do not be ignorant of the kleshas (afflictions).

Practice discrimination. Understand the mind, understand the soul. The mind is effected by the Gunas, the Soul is beyond that.

2.27

The knowledge is sevenfold:

You are in tune with your body and understand the Gunas and how you can leave them behind, becoming in touch with the soul.

You realize you are spirit in a physical body.

You learn from your challenges in life.

You learn to control the mind.

You will have self-realizations.

There will be absence of suffering.

You know the self, you understand your soul purpose.

2.28

Through your spiritual practice you reach a state of clarity of the mind, a healthy body and a wise soul. These are the gifts and freedoms of your hard work and effort.

See your wisdom shine through.

Wear the golden crown of power and enlightenment.

2.29

Patanjali's eight limbs of Yoga, known as Ashtanga Yoga, are:

Yama - code of conduct)

Niyama - attitude to yourself) life vows

Asana - postures

Pranayama - breathing techniques

Pratyahara - withdrawal of the senses, going within

Dharana - concentration

Dyhana - meditation

Samadhi - enlightenment

The eight limbs are the structural framework of Yoga practice.

2.30

The five Yamas are as follows:

Ahimsa - non-violence

Satya - the truth, right speech
Asteya - not stealing, having integrity
Brahmacarya - moderation
Aparigrahah - non-greed

2.31

It doesn't matter what background you have, what culture you come from, these vows should be practiced by everyone, particularly for those actively on their spiritual paths. You are being made aware of these principles, through study of the texts and/or your Teacher.

2.32

Yamas are universal life skills and the Niyamas are for the individual self.
The five Niyamas are:
Sauca - cleanliness, purity
Santosa - being content
Tapas - self-discipline
Svadhyaya - self-study
Isvara pranidhanani - connecting to The Great Divine

2.33

Yamas and Niyamas are similar to the ten commandments and are guides and disciplines towards our selves and others. They are common-sense guidelines of how to lead a healthier, happier life - bringing spiritual awareness into a social context. It is good spiritual practice to question, challenge and contemplate these guidelines and put them into context with our everyday lives and resonate with them, discover our own truths. To study the Yamas and Niyamas will help us to manage our energy in a positive way, to contemplate our outer life with our own inner development. They help us to view ourselves and others with compassion and awareness. They help us to respect others' values and they help us to lead a conscious life.

Different challenges will be put to us as we travel through life and it is how we react and deal with these challenges that matter so that we can evolve and grow as a human being.

The Planet would be in love, peace and harmony if these ten codes of conduct were practiced by all.

2.34

Think of the consequences of your actions.

These actions could be in the form of speech - do not harm yourself or others with your words - be careful what you say.

These actions could be in the form of physical - before taking action in life, think of the outcome. Do not physically harm yourself or others - the outcome will only cause more problems.

2.35

Yamas - codes of conduct - 1ˢᵗ limb of Ashtanga Yoga
Ahimsa - non-violence

Ahimsa is non-violence, non-injury, kindness, no harm in your actions. Awareness and gentleness in action, thought and speech. Violence arises out of fear, anger, restlessness and selfishness. We should practice compassion, love, under-standing, patience, self-love and worthiness.

To apply this to ourselves we should keep our mind healthy and positive which in turn will have a positive effect on our bodies and soul.

If you don't think harmful thoughts, then your whole energy system will be much lighter and will attract non-harmful thinking people. If you hold harmful thoughts then this can be sensed by others by being in your presence and for those that really see, in your aura.

Another thought on ahimsa is not to harm any animals. To some this will mean not to eat meat and become a vegetarian or certainly if you do eat meat then be mindful, to only purchase free-range, freedom food and not that from a factory farm where the poor animal has suffered misery from the second they are born to the second they are slaughtered. Also, why buy meat from animals that have traveled in inhumane conditions across many countries when you can buy local? Imagine the energy and suffering that will affect the meat that is then going into your body. A good practice is to bless your food before eating or say a prayer giving thanks to the animal.

Be mindful.

Animals have their own levels of consciousness and it is beyond comprehension how a human being can be cruel to animals and allow them to suffer.

2.36

Satya - truthfulness - of speech, thoughts and deeds

Right speech means speaking what is true, useful and beneficial, pleasant and gentle, timely, friendly and kind. Right speech means refraining from: Telling lies, gossiping, saying harsh things about others, abusive language.

Speak your own truths. As you walk along your spiritual path you learn to speak from the heart and not straight from the head.

2.37

Asteya - not stealing

Do not take from others what is not yours. Live with integrity and sleep well at night knowing that you have not hurt others or taken anything from them.

Treat others how you would like to be treated yourself. Gain confidence from others, knowing that they can trust you.

Remember the laws of karma - if you take from others, in time others will take from you tenfold.

2.38

Bramacarya - moderation, self-containment

Do not overindulge the mind, intellect, speech or body; moderation on all levels concerning sex, food and all aspects of daily life including the environment.

We should practice not repression, but control of sensual cravings. Years ago Yogis in India would have abstained from sex. They believed that by suppressing sexual energy this would channel everything into their spiritual practice. Moderation would be more appropriate to us "House-holder" Yogis!

Moderation can be applied to alcohol also. It is not easy in modern times to totally give up sex, alcohol, meat, sugar etc so moderation is the key.

2.39

Aparigraha - non-greed

Being content with what you have will make you a happy and fulfilled person. Don't hanker after more than you need which is greed. Have what you need around you and don't get carried away with wanting more and more - know when to stop.

Apply this to possessions, food, money, ambitions.

Only take what you need.

Keep it real.

2.40

Niyamas - attitude to ourselves - 2nd limb of Ashtanga Yoga

How we interact with ourselves, our internal world.

Sauca - purity, cleanliness

The physical exterior body should be kept cleansed every day with water.

The body can be cleansed internally firstly with the correct diet, having knowledge of a good balanced diet, and by drinking plenty of water.

Practicing asana and pranayama is cleansing to the energy

system of the body and will help to remove toxins and impurities.

Your own home should be kept clean and tidy.

2.40

This will result in a tidy mind.

2.41

Santosa - contentment

Accept what is, make the best out of everything. Being content brings you joy and happiness.

Being free from desires is being at peace.

Being discontented leads to a restless soul.

2.43

Tapas - self-discipline

The willingness to do what is necessary to reach a goal with discipline. This could mean making sacrifices in certain areas and having the determination to pursue daily practices. Tapas actually means "heat" or "fire" - go through the heat and accept it - invite it in. The fire brings transformation - burn off some layers and emerge as something new. Long sitting meditation is a disciplined practice - physical heat is generated, which "burns" the ego away to reveal the true inner spirit.

We need self-discipline with our spiritual practice; we need to do asana, pranayama and meditation regularly. We also need discipline with what we eat and drink - take food that we know and feel is good for our body and provides us with the necessary nutrition - not too much, not too little.

2.44

Svadhyaya - study of the self

By studying sacred texts and observing the self over time, you will realize the self.

Svadhyaya is the study of sacred texts of all religions and philosophies and finding what resonates with you. Also the study of ourselves, who we are, what we are and why we behave as we do!

This means to look inside oneself, to study oneself. This is about considering the meaning of spiritual concepts - understanding the underlying wisdom, not accepting without question. Expand knowledge through reading, study the scriptures and relate them to the self and to life.

It is useful when you are ready to seek a teacher or healer who can help you find the essence of who you truly are, someone who is working at a soul level.

2.45

Isvarapranidhana - devotion to an ideal, to The Great Divine, surrender

We all have a need to realize the TRUTH and meaning of life.

To practice faith, dedication, sincerity and patience to transcend the ego, which is so resistant to surrender.

Isvarapranidhana is about our relationship to the Great Divine Energy of the Universe. It is about communing with this Energy - God - The Great Spirit - realizing that this Spirit is within us and that we are part of it - we are all one.

You can connect with the Universe by prayer, through meditation, through repeating Mantra.

Trust with The Great Divine and know you are being heard, feel the pure divine love that is around you, surrender.

Be in Samadhi.

2.46

Asana - posture - 3rd limb of Ashtanga Yoga

Asana translates as 'posture' the word derives from the Sanskrit root 'as' which means 'to stay', 'to be', 'to sit' or 'to be established in a particular position'.

Patanjali's Yoga Sutra describes an asana as having two important qualities: sthira and sukha. Sthira is steadiness and alertness, Sukha refers to the ability to remain comfortable in a posture. Both qualities should be present to the same degree when practising any posture.

The postures have three steps, first is taking the position, second is the Asana or position itself and third is releasing the position. It is necessary that the movement involved should be slow and steady, you should avoid fast movement, jerks, strains and the locking out of joints.

Asana will improve your strength and flexibility.

To learn the postures it is best to go to a qualified teacher.

Be focused when practicing the postures and work with the breath. Dharana (concentration) begins with Asana.

If any postures do not feel right or you feel like you are straining, then come out of the posture with care and attention.

2.47

Do not fight the postures. Let go and feel the postures. Focus on the breath, on the movement and where in the body you feel the energy.

Let go.

Energy will shift in the body, toxins will be released. This is often subtle, but very powerful.

2.48

You start to feel unity of energies, you connect to your body. You will have the ability to tune into your physical body, feel the energy within, know where you have blocked energy and understand when the body is healthy.

When perfection in a posture is gained, the mind, body and spirit become one.

Dualities do not exist any more, only unity.

2.49
Pranayama - breathing - 4th limb of Ashtanga Yoga

Prana is energy.

Observe your breathing.

Watch the inhale, watch the exhale.

See that there is a natural pause after the inhale and after the exhale.

Breathe to the full length of your breath.

Inhale pure energy, exhale impurities.

Everything around you is energy - things you see such as people, animals, plants.

There are energy centers below you, above you and within you.

The seven main centers within are known as the Chakras. These centers form the subtle body.

2.50

Retention of the breath is known as kumbhaka.

Retention after the inhale is known as antara kumbhaka.

Retention after the exhale is known as bahya kumbhaka.

An example would be:

Inhale for count of 6

Hold for count of 3 (antara kumbhaka)

Exhale for count of 6

Hold for count of 3 (bahya kumbhaka)

The mind is then fixed on the breath and is in preparation for Meditation.

When the breath is still, everything is still.

2.51

Focus on an external object whilst observing the breath.

Visualize yourself standing on a beach. Focus on your breathing.

Observe your inhale, pause. Observe your exhale, pause.

As you inhale see the wave coming into the shore, pause.

As you exhale, see the wave going back out to the sea, pause.

Repeat several times.

Bring yourself back by focusing on just the breath, feel the abdomen rising on the inhale, falling on the exhale.

2.52

Be free.

Discover real peace.

2.53

Your mind becomes empty.

You are ready to enter the gateway to Dharana - concentration.

2.54

Pratyahara - going inwards - 5th limb of Ashtanga Yoga

The mind has discovered peace. Attention is focused.

Out of your head space and into your Self.

The five senses withdraw and go within.

There are no desires or attachments, the ego deflates. Vairagya is the practice of non-attachment and renunciation.

Imagine Pratyahara in the form of a huge Oak tree. The trunk of the tree is hollowed out for you to enter and go down into the earth - going into the self.

2.55

Once you go into this tree and down into the earth - you will enter into the Soul.

Chapter 3

Vibhuti Pada – The Magic Powers

Chapter III starts by explaining the last three limbs of Patanjali's eight limbs of Yoga (Ashtanga Yoga) - Dharana (concentration), Dhyana (Meditation) and Samadhi (beautiful blissful state) and how the three integrate into Samyana.

Here we learn of the siddhis which are the supernatural powers that are a gift to those who connect to The Great Divine. However, there is a warning that this gift could come at a cost - further progress to your spiritual practice. It is easy to become distracted by these powers; this is a lesson in ego. Some people connect deeply to their Spiritual Guides or to Angels for instance, however there is a warning to not become too attached to these guides and celestial beings, this is not liberation. You may have beautiful experiences connecting with these allies, but this is not the goal. True transformation takes place when you have a shift in energy, this cannot be attained through the siddhis.

This shift in energy can be attained through your continued effort to work with your energy, getting to know and understand the esoteric body. Understanding the chakras and connecting deeply with the self will allow healing to take place.

3.1

Dharana - concentration - 6th limb of Ashtanga Yoga

Dharana (sixth limb of Ashtanga Yoga), is being totally focused on one object - concentrated attention. This object could be either within the body i.e.: focusing on one of the chakras (energy centers within), or on the breath, or outside the body which could be a statue of an icon, for example, such as Buddha, a picture of your Spiritual Teacher. The object could also be in the form of words; a Mantra. Repetition of a Mantra directed to The Great Divine will completely engage the mind. An example of a Mantra is OM MANI PADME HUM - the Buddhist chant of compassion.

3.2

Dhyana - meditation - 7th limb of Ashtanga Yoga

Dhyana is the seventh limb of Ashtanga Yoga. This stage is where the mind stays focused on this object for some length of time - this is meditation. The mind stays concentrated just on the object and time stays still.

3.3

Samadhi - 8th limb of Ashtanga Yoga

All awareness is on the object. Dhyana will flow into Samadhi once all attention is upon the object with no distractions and no self-awareness. This is truly a blissful state.

Craftsmen experience a level of Samadhi when they are putting all their focus into their work, concentrating just on what they are doing, with the mind just being in the present. For example, a Stone Mason as he is working on carving the stone with his mind being on just what he is doing at that moment in time.

However, Craftsmen who need to have their attention very focused may only get a glimpse of Samadhi as their attention is not sustained. Whereas the person who actively aims for this state can sustain Samadhi.

It is an incredibly peaceful and beautiful place to be.

3.4

Samyama - integration of dharana (concentration), Dyhana (meditation) and Samadhi (beautiful blissful state).

When the mind is fully concentrated (dharana) but you are still aware of where you are, sitting in a room, perhaps focusing on an object such as Buddha. You then go into meditation (dhyana). There are no distractions, just total focus, showing perfect inner discipline. The next level of consciousness is then achieved and is sustained (Samadhi) that beautiful blissful state. One follows the other and you become at one with the object.

3.5

You may experience 'light-bulb' moments as you journey along your path - moments of illumination and self-awareness. You may get a realization on an issue, something from the past or something that you needed guidance on, something that may be troubling your mind. These light-bulb moments is you connecting to your soul, the voice of intuition is being heard.
Your own wisdoms will shine through, you may feel elated.

3.6

Use these insights wisely. Listen to your voice that is now heard. This is not knowledge that can be read from books, this is pure wisdom, the higher truth.

3.7

Try different techniques of meditation. See sutras 1.27, 1.35, 1.36, 1.37, 1.41 and 2.51.

Dharana, Dhyana and Samadhi are seen as internal aspects of Yoga. These involve going in to the self. The Yamas and Niyamas are the Universal laws of conduct. Asana focuses the attention on the physical body through posture work.

Pranayama focuses the attention to the breath - the inhale, the exhale, prana the life force. Pratyahara is where the five senses start to quieten down and withdraw so the concept of going inwards begins.

3.8

Once you reach Samadhi and are connected as one energy with The Great Divine, you are One.
You are no longer "in" the self. "You" are no longer.
You are in beauty with Spirit.

3.9

When we are distracted our breathing becomes heavier and irregular. When we are concentrated our breathing becomes lighter and quiet, we are absorbed in our meditation, in a very serene state.

3.10

It is beautiful for the mind, body and spirit to be really still, in a tranquil state - peace.
Much practice is required to still the mind.

3.11

Be in peace, in Samadhi, be still and allow this transformation to happen, naturally.

3.12

The transformation can only take place if this focused attention is maintained. If you put too much effort in and are trying too hard your awareness will come and go from being aware to unaware.

3.13

Changes will take place within the mind, body and spirit.

Energy will shift. It is so subtle, yet powerful.

3.14
Don't try and analyze what these changes are - just be with this. You may get realizations today, tomorrow or next week - don't hold on - just process the thoughts and let it go.

3.15
Think of this transformation taking place like a snake shedding its skin. This is you shedding old energy from the past, ready for your next cycle.

3.16
You will see things differently, for the better.
Psychic powers can develop. There is a word of warning not to allow these powers (Siddhis) to act as a distraction from your spiritual path. You may see the past and sometimes the future. You may be able to see this in others, this could be a burden not only to you but to the other person who may not be ready to know.

3.17
Practice Samyana (integration of Dharana, Dhyana and Samadhi) on sound.
This sound can be a word, an animal calling, or sound from a musical instrument.
Try using an image of an animal as your object of concentration. Call in this animal, feel the energy, what can this offer you? What is this energy you need at the present time? Get to know your Power Animal, it is your ally. Feel like you are this animal, hear the sounds.
For example, as you sit in meditation, call in your Power Animal, your ally. See this friend - a beautiful Hawk appears to you. The Hawk has incredible eyes - to give you clear vision. It

misses nothing with these eyes - it sees everything clearly. It's energy feels very bright and alert. See the world through the eyes of the Hawk. It's call is piercing. It is short but sharp, that energy can be used in speech - be heard, get straight to the point, speak your truths.

3.18

We may start to see past lives and how they can help us with this life.

We may see our bloodline as we journey back through our ancestors. See the beautiful gifts they have given to us and also the limitations and challenges.

3.19

We become more self-aware. We correct our posture often during the course of the day and our posture is improved. We observe our behaviour - how we deal with different emotions such as anger, when the blood feels like it is boiling and the breath gets faster, we learn to control our emotions.

You may start to see others as they really are. It may not be possible to actually read another's mind but you may be able to assess their state of mind. You may be able to read their energy, look into their aura. For example if you see red in their aura, it could mean they are passionate, or possibly angry. If you see pink, it could mean they are in a good space with love - they love themselves and give their love to others. If you see purple, this could mean they are healers.

3.20

It could be potentially damaging to tell others what you see in them as they may not be ready to be healed. For example, if you feel they have an illness of the digestive system then what is the point in telling them something they already know? If you feel that they have cancer in their body, then you are faced with a dilemma. You mention it so they can consult a medic, but by getting it wrong you may frighten them half to death.

3.21

The subtle body is sometimes known as the esoteric body which means the energy system within us, our chakras and around us, our aura.
Being in touch with the subtle body is an amazing gift.

3.22

This gift should be used wisely.

3.23

Practice Samyana on your past lives. Your vision may become so clear that you may be able to see your own past and future and the time of your own death in this life.

3.24

Practice Samyana on various kinds of strength such as physical, mental, moral, psychic and spiritual and see your power grow.
During your life there may have been incidents, challenges, possible traumas. These may have been a shock to your system causing you to lose part of your energy at that moment - your life force. By observing these incidents, you can bring back your life force. Sometimes it is good practice to actually see your energy returning, then the real healing can take place.

3.25

Let your focus be on your life force.
Let your power be strong.
Walk in your own power.

3.26

Clairsentience may develop as the energy in your heart gets

stronger, feelings are intensified.

Clairaudience may develop as the energy around your throat centre increases - communication - speech, ears for listening.

Clairvoyance will develop as your brow centre (Ajna) is cleared and you may start to see, with the eyes closed.

3.27

Samyana on the Cosmos - the Sun, the Moon, the Stars and Planets.

Surya - the Sun

The Sun energy is related to the Male within us. On a physical level, it corresponds to our sympathetic nervous system. Our male energy is our ego which is connected to our self-esteem and confidence. The Sun is the fire energy within us, this is represented by the Spirit. It is believed that Samyana on the Sun, will give us "knowledge of the seven worlds"; the seven chakras within our body that are located down the spine.

There are also several chakras below us and several above our Crown. Chakra means wheel of energy.

The base chakra is usually seen as an earthy red/brown colour and is known as the Mooladhara. This word means "root". It is situated at the very base of the body.

The sacral chakra is usually seen as an orange energy and is known as Svadhistana. It is situated below the navel.

The solar plexus chakra is usually seen as a bright yellow and is known as Manipura. It is situated around the stomach area.

The heart chakra is usually seen as a beautiful green or pink energy and is known as Anahata. It is situated around the heart area.

The throat chakra is usually seen as a blue energy. It is known as Visuddha. It is situated around the throat area.

The brow chakra is usually seen as indigo or purple energy and is known as Ajna. It is situated above the nose around the brow area.

The crown chakra is usually seen as white or violet or gold energy and is known as Sahasrara - the thousand petalled lotus flower. It is situated on the top of the head.

3.28
Chandra - The Moon
Samyana on The Moon will get us in touch with our feminine side.
The Moon energy within us is our feminine, goddess energy. Whereas the solar plexus is linked to the Sun, the lunar plexus which is situated in the cerebrum is linked to The Moon. She is our intuitive side, our unconscious and is linked to the element of water - our emotions, this energy corresponds to our parasympathetic nervous system on a physical level, our calming energy.
The cycle of the Moon is the same length of time as the female menstrual cycle - 28 days. The Moon has three phases - waxing, full and waning. The Moon at one time was worshipped as a powerful force and her energy effects water tides. The planting of seeds and crops would have been done at a certain phase of the Moon, as well as harvesting.

3.29
Samyana on the Cosmos - the Stars, the Planets. This will bring you great insight. Imagine the knowledge that Astrologers have of the planets and how they can draw up birth charts which tell you so much about yourself and what energies you are working with.
However, nothing is written in stone and through life you have free will to make your own choices.

3.30
The next few sutras mention Samyana on particular parts of the body.

By Samyana on the naval, you will gain knowledge of your body - your digestive system, your organs, your heart, your breathing. You will get to know when there is a blockage of energy which could possibly lead to a physical problem.

Get to know your esoteric body - your chakras and nadis (channels of energy also known as meridians). Be in tune with your energy.

3.31

By Samyana on the throat you will get to understand how you communicate. How do you speak? Fast, as you have so much to say that you can't get it out quick enough? Loud, as you liked to be heard? Are you too quiet and suppress what you want to say? Are you a good listener? When someone talks, are you listening or are you already thinking of the next thing to say?

3.32

By Samyana on the hollow below the throat you feel the whole body relaxing, becoming very quiet and still.

3.33

By Samyana just above the Crown you may start to see the spirit world which means:

Loved ones in spirit

Spirit Guides - those in light who come to you to guide and protect

Earthlings - faeries, elves and little earth beings

Angels and Archangels

Ascended Masters

Spirit will only link to you when you are ready. Spirit can link to you through the practice of meditation and active awareness.

Spirit can come through on any of the above dimensions depending on what level you are on - this depends on your self and your own development and awareness, your studies, your wisdom. Spirit will only link to you if your intentions are pure; for guidance and support to the self and those in need.

3.34

All the hidden knowledge is revealed. You have discovered the golden key and you have unlocked true wisdom.

3.35

By Samyana on the heart, your true self will emerge.
Instead of being led by the ego, you will be led by intuition.

3.36

The soul has been here before in many past lives. The mind has not.

3.37

You are spirit in a physical body.
Around your body is your energy field. Your chakras are linked to this energy field with vibrations. All around you is energy, spirit, light. As you peel off your layers of blocked emotions and negative thoughts, your energy field expands and becomes clear of these blockages; your light gets brighter. Your chakras will shine like beautiful jewels.
The individual self becomes whole. Your lower chakras link to the earth energies and your upper chakras (from the heart upwards) link to spirit energies. Your sense of seeing, taste, hearing, touching and smelling develops. In time these senses will be used not only on the earth plane but when you are linked in to the spirit plane.

3.38

There is a warning here that these powers can be an obstacle to your spiritual path. The ego could easily get caught up in the power that these gifts bring. Also, you may think that this is the ultimate goal; seeing spirit, hearing spirit, smelling in the spirit world. They are however a distraction to the true path of self-realization and enlightenment. It is not enlightenment to see the pretty colours of the chakras - this is opening of awareness. It is not a party trick you use to impress others when you can see their auras, feel their illness or tell them their destiny. (How potentially damaging can that be)?

Some may have these gifts brought to them very early on in life and this can be seen as a hindrance. There are Psychics who claim "they were born a Clairvoyant" - they see spirit and give messages to others from lost loved ones in spirit. These are gifts that all can tap into. Although that said, some are clearly here to work with these gifts to heal others pain.

Do not get attached to these powers do not allow them to inflate your ego. However do not be fearful of them or pretend they don't exist. Just acknowledge this is part of your spiritual growth. You can then move forward along your spiritual path towards Kaivalya - liberation.

3.39

Once you understand and have mastered the concept of the esoteric body - the chakras and energy system, great healing and transformation can take place. If it is your destiny and your gift, you can start teaching and healing others by working with their energy system. Therapies such as Reiki are brilliant for spreading knowledge of the esoteric body and show that by laying the hands in the aura or on the physical body how energy can be channelled.

3.40

Vayu means air. There are five main energy functions and these are: apana, samana, prana, udana and vyana.

Apana

Apana is the energy in the area of the body of the lower abdomen and controls the functioning of the kidneys, colon and rectum, the bladder and genitals. So apana energy is concerned with the function of elimination.

Samana

Samana is the energy in the stomach area of the body and controls the function of digestion and metabolism. Samana also activates the heart and circulatory system and is responsible for the assimilation and distribution of nutrients.

Prana

Prana is the energy around the chest region. It affects speech and the vocal cords, and the respiratory system. Through Prana Vayu we are able to absorb energy from our food and drink and from the air around us - through the skin, tongue and of course through breathing.

Udana

Udana is energy around the throat area and effects the function of speech - expression and communication.

Vyana

Vyana effects the distribution of energy into all areas of the body. It regulates and controls all movement, and coordinates the other pranas. It acts as the reserve energy for the other pranas.

3.41

By Samyana on the vayus, your body will radiate light.

3.42

By Samyana on the link between space (ether) and sound, the

gift of clairaudience will be given. You will hear the sounds that others will not hear.

3.43

You will feel as light as a feather. You understand the sensation of floating, of levitating.

3.44

You feel like you are floating on a cloud.

3.45

By Samyana on the elements, you will become Master over them all.

These five elements are fire, water, earth, air and ether. These elements are forms of energy. Everything in nature relates to these elements including us - we all have parts of these energies within us.

We need the element of fire to keep our spirit alive.

We need the element of water for our emotions.

We need the element of earth to keep us grounded.

We need the element of air for our minds, our mental energy.

We need the element of ether to connect us to space.

Your birth sign will show what energy is strongest and weakest in you. For example, a Cancerian is a Water sign so emotional energy is strong in this sign. Cancerians are in .touch with their feelings.

Gemini is an air sign and you often find Geminis have very active mental energy - they find it particularly difficult to calm their mind.

Aries - fire

Taurus - earth

Gemini - air

Cancer - water

Leo - fire

Virgo - earth
Libra - air
Scorpio - water
Sagittarius - fire
Capricorn - earth
Aquarius - air
Pisces - water

You may find it useful as part of self-study (svadhyaya) to discover what energies are in your chart.

3.46

You can get in tune with the self by focusing on these elements:

Visualization:

Visualize yourself walking along a sandy beach. Feel the sand coming up between your toes. The sun is shining down upon you. Stop and lie down on the sand. Feel the energy of the sun - Fire. How does it feel?

You get up from the sand and look at the ocean. It is still, like a pond. Step into the water and feel the coolness over your feet. The water is crystal clear. How do you feel connecting to the element of water?

You go back on to the beach and turn around and ahead of you is a path. Go to the path and walk slowly up. The path takes you up a hill and ahead of you is a gate. Go through the gate and enter a landscape of beautiful lush green countryside. There are trees, wild flowers and wild animals. Feel the connection to Mother Earth with every step you take. How does it feel to be connected to the element of earth?

You feel a cool breeze and look up and see the trees swaying. You are alone in this beautiful landscape. You breathe in the fresh air filling your lungs, taking long slow deep breaths. Feel the connection of the element of air. How does it feel?

You look up to the sky. It is a beautiful pale blue. Breathe in this vast open space. Feel yourself being taken up to the clouds. Feel

ether. How does it feel?
Slowly bring yourself back to the present,
Ground yourself to finish.

3.47
Be in the beauty of these elements.

3.48
Be in the beauty of nature.
Let go of the ego.
Just be.

3.49
Understand the elements and understand the self.

3.50
See the soul.

3.51
Be free.
Renounce the siddhis - the supernatural powers. Don't become attached to them, as they then become an obstacle to the true spiritual path.
The siddhis are there to attain Samadhi. Use them when you need them, be mindful with the right intent.

3.52
Do not become attached to your Spirit Guides and friends.
You may be tempted to be in awe when your Spirit Guides, Angels, Archangels, Friends come to you. Do not be in awe, you are in your power and these are your allies but you must not let them become a distraction or you will not be able to progress on your path.

3.53
Learn to live with awareness. Take this into your daily life.
Acknowledge special awareness moments. This is the true
beauty of living.
For example, when you are away on holiday leaving the routine
of your daily life behind, your mind becomes focused on the
moment. This is much easier when you are away from the
pressures that having a job, home and family can bring. You
have freedom to do what you want, when you want. You are the
boss, calling the shots. When you are swimming in the sea, your
mind will be in the present because that is all you have to worry
about - the water, your swimming.

When you return home to your everyday life, do not let your
mind go back to its old habits of running away, moaning to you
about the pressures of getting up in the morning, going back to
work, be aware of where you are at the present moment.

Your allies are there for you to call upon when you need them.
There will be times when discrimination is required between
your needs and your habits.

3.54
Allow yourself time for reflection. Self-realizations can only be
found if your mind has space. Spend time alone when you can.
It is helpful to find a quiet "sit-spot" in nature; a place where
you cannot be disturbed such as a space in the forest, find a log
to sit on.

3.55
Sacred knowledge cannot be read in books or held in the intelligence. It is something that you have always known deep within
but have not accessed before. When your truth is revealed, you
will feel an energy emerging from deep within. It is like coming
home.

3.56

Be in Kaivalya - be liberated.

Free.

Chapter 4

Kaivalya Pada – Freedom and Liberation

Your spiritual practice is a continuous journey. Kaivalya is freedom - emancipation - liberation; from suffering, from the afflictions, you will have learnt how to let go of your wounds and past issues.

Chapter four is like giving you a 'pat on the back' saying well done for coming this far, but don't give up your practice, your journey has not ended. Incorporate what you have learnt into your daily life. You will experience wonderful meditation and possibly out of body experiences but you cannot be in this place 'twenty four seven'. Be in both worlds - have your feet on the ground, and be connected with Spirit.

You have learnt to walk in your own power and you understand the concept of mind, body and soul. You know the self, you have done much work and you walk and live in light. Your healing will show in the way you speak, walk and show yourself to the world. Others will feel your beautiful presence and your healing energies will spread to others and out to the Universe.

Once you become a clear channel (through self development and healing your wounds), you may become a spiritual teacher yourself. Pass what you have learnt on to others.

4.1

There are five main ways for you to achieve spiritual power:

Being born with these powers.

Through the use of herbs or drugs.

Chanting mantras.

Devotional practice.

Meditation.

Being born with these powers: we all have the capabilities to tap into the siddhis (spiritual powers). There are certain people who have these gifts from birth to use to help others. It could be said that these are a gift or the fruits of previous lives. Some may see them as a burden. (To see spirit as a child could be a frightening experience). Others have inherited these gifts from their ancestors.

Through the use of herbs or drugs: many people today think they can fast-track their spiritual experiences by taking drugs to experience hallucination. This is a temporary insight that can be very damaging. (There are natural herbs that can be taken such as Ayahuasca in Peru which can be seen by some as spiritually cleansing).

Chanting mantras: by chanting sacred words and repeating them quietens the mind and can lead to the senses withdrawing, taking you into deep contemplation.

Devotional practice: tapas; self-discipline to get you to practice daily. This may be in the form of energy work - exercise, Yoga postures, Tai Chi. Continued self-study; you have come so far with contemplating the self, now you may be ready to do some soul work; to work at a deeper level with the self.

Meditation; you will have practiced different techniques and now you should know what works for you.

4.2

Your practice is becoming more powerful. You find you can meditate easier. Your mind is more disciplined. You are connected to nature. You understand the concept of being grounded but also being connected to spirit.

4.3

You are in touch with your esoteric body - you own energy system. You can feel grounding energies in your lower chakras. You can also feel connected to spirit from your upper chakras. Your energy does not leak out, it flows beautifully like a river.

4.4

You learn to channel energy correctly. If someone tries to anger you, you don't hold onto this anger, you let it go. The tyrants around you - those that are judgmental, critical, racist, opinionated no longer bother you. You have learnt to not take on any energy that is harmful to your mind and your spirit.

4.5

You are learning to be led by your intuition; the truth, rather than by the ego; the distorted truth.
Follow your heart.

4.6

Meditation will diminish the shadow self. Emotions such as lust, greed, fear, jealousy and anger will be subdued.
Your mind learns to let go.

4.7

An accomplished Yogi does not get caught up in the dramas of life. They are beyond that. Simplicity is the key. Apply this to your daily practice; keep your posture practice simple, do your breathing being mindful and don't try and make your meditations too elaborate. Also apply this to your life - don't make life complicated. If you are tired and feel that you are doing too much, don't fill your diary up with appointments. If you have a good Yoga class to go to in your local area, avoid the one that is an hour away. Give yourself some free time, have some peace and quiet - turn off the television, the radio, the telephone.

Even Yoga can become an attachment. As you do your daily practice you should be mindful, not wishing you were somewhere else, you should be in a lovely present, peaceful place. You should enjoy your practice because you know the benefits it brings to you. Your motives and desires should be pure; with the right intent. Spiritual practice should be regular but should not become a chore.

When practicing postures, do them because you want to be doing them, not because you have to. If your mind is continually resisting that day, then stop and go and do something else, then perhaps come back when you are ready.

4.8

In your past lives you may have been a man or you may have been a woman.

If it is your belief, your soul may have had an animal incarnation. You may find that you are drawn to a particular animal and the energy of that animal can teach you certain lessons in this life and bring certain energies to you.

4.9

Karmic lessons will come to you at the right time in your life. If you do not learn from these lessons, they will come to you repeatedly until you "see". You are likely to have had past lives with those closest to you. Often our family members are our best "teachers".

Desires and attachments are often seeds from past lives. For example, you can never seem to settle where you are. You always want to move. You spend your live moving home and after a few years, you want to move again. Each time you move, the desire returns. This is a good situation to look into a past life where you may discover you were part of a Nomadic tribe who were continually moving and this seed is planted within you but comes in the form of a desire that cannot be fulfilled.

4.10
Your soul chose this life, whether you are male or female, your race, culture and environment. Your soul wishes to become whole so it can ascend, becoming a Spirit Guide, Helper, Teacher, Master, and from there help earth beings to become whole also.

4.11
Through your spiritual work, the soul will find liberation from earthly energies; attachments and desires. Obstacles will be removed through practice, the Gunas no longer exist, karma will be released through your effort and awareness. Kaivalya (freedom, liberation, emancipation) will be truly experienced.
No more desires.
Freedom from suffering.
Letting go of past wounds and issues.
No more afflictions.

4.12
Your wounds will be healed. Your mind does not cling to the Kleshas. (Avidya - spiritual unawareness, asmita - ego, raga - attachments, dvesha - hatred, anger and abhinivesa - fears). Your dramas are over.
You will not be ruled by time, for you there is no time, there just is.

4.13
You can now live with this freedom. You are out of the dark and live in light. You still have your earthly duties - your family, your work but you are above all the dramas that exist around

you. You have been working at a deep soul level. You have recognised the gifts and freedoms that your family have given you and you have also worked on the limitations and burdens. You see the lessons that life has thrown at you. You have true wisdom and are very knowing. This is Kaivalya.

4.14

You exist in a Sattvic state - in luminosity. You understand the pitfalls of being in tamasic energies (heavy, inertia). You understand rajasic energies (overly energetic).

You apply this to your mind, body and spirit.

4.15

You have found your way with your spiritual path. You know what feels right to you, what energies you are comfortable with. You know what meditation techniques work for you.

You have found what is sacred to you and you understand that what are your beliefs and truths are not necessarily another's beliefs and truths. You have respect for all others' places of worship and their deity, for you have found yours.

You understand the concept of being true to who you are. You connect with the energies in your culture, in your environment. For example, if you are born in Great Britain, then connect to the beautiful Goddess energy, connect to sacred sites that you feel at home with. Have a "sit-spot" out in nature - somewhere like in a forest, or in a field or in a park near a tree, where you can sit quietly and connect to nature.

This doesn't mean to say not to explore other ways - other cultures have beautiful spiritual ceremonies such as the Native American Indians (like The Vision Quest - going off into nature alone for days with very little to eat and drink and waiting for spirit to come), but be who you really are.

4.16

There will be a certain level of consciousness because we have to go about our daily lives. We can't all live in caves seeking spiritual solace or become Sadhus (wandering spiritual seekers in India). However, it is possible to live our lives being in awareness. If we went about our lives in a constant blissful state with our head in the clouds, then we wouldn't have the grounding energies to go to work, look after our families and pay the bills. This is where we learn to balance our spiritual life with our earthly life and live in harmony.

Learn to live with awareness.

4.17

You will become free from your conditioning. Your conditioning is your environment from the past - how you were brought up, the rules and regulations in your society.

Your perception will allow you to take what you can take from your upbringing (conditioning from family, schools, friends) and what you can leave behind.

4.18

The true self is the soul - the seer - Perusha.

It is the Lord and Master - of the mind.

4.19

The mind then exists through the soul. You will gain access to the higher truths.

4.20

It is not possible for the mind to exist through the ego and the soul at the same time.

4.21

Consciousness is one.

4.22

Your consciousness will be raised and you will have access to other dimensions. The mind has attained purity. The body is cleansed and the spirit within is connected.

4.23

We Are All One Consciousness.

4.24

You will no longer confuse the mind as the master.

4.25

You have now reached the highest state of clarity.
You will not be distracted by tyrants, afflictions and sufferings.

4.26

Liberation is attained.

4.27

Continued practice must take place as it is possible to regress back to states of confusion and go back into old patterns of behavior. Discernment is required.

4.28

All the work of ridding yourself of the afflictions; the five kleshas - avidya, asmita, raga, dvesha, abhinivesa, will be rewarded with bliss, peace, balance and harmony. You should still be aware that regression is possible.
You will never stop learning in life.

4.29

You feel the beauty of life. You see and feel the beauty of nature. Your inner light is so bright that you glow. Others will feel this in your presence. You feel Divine Love.

4.30

You are free from Karma and the Kleshas - the afflictions.
There is no more suffering.

4.31

Now you are walking in your own power. You do not quote
from books or from teachers, you speak from your heart. You
know your truths and you are now wisdom itself.

4.32

You are love and light.

4.33

You are free from the gunas - you are in the light.
You have reached self-realization.
You are at one with The Great Divine.

4.34

You are pure consciousness.
Kaivalya - liberation.

Summary

The main points to focus on to help you on your spiritual quest are:

Moving energy in the form of physical movement which can be in the form of Yoga Postures.

To practice forms of breathing techniques. To focus on the breath, to learn to breathe using full capacity of the lungs.

To practice meditation - trying the various types of techniques such as focusing on the breath, using visualizations, working with sound - musical instruments, chanting.

To practice Svadhyaya - self-study and study of sacred texts. Work on healing your wounds, peel off the layers that have built up over the years developing patterns, holding on to the past, learn to let go. Learn from your challenges and lessons in life.

Be free, at peace, happy and healthy.

Thanks

I would like to firstly thank The Masters in Spirit who helped me with this book, my Spirit Allies and the following Earth Allies: my beautiful family, my Great Teachers who are Swami Satchidananda Mataji, Trudi Morgan, Carol Holly, Gilly Towers, Eagle's Wing - Dawn Russell and Lorraine Grayston and my other Great Teachers - my students, from whom I have learnt so much.

Some of the royalties of this book will go towards the following charities:
Satchidananda Wholistic Trust (will go to Orphanage in Rishikesh, Omkarananda Ashram) and Sivananda Ashram
Crisis - homeless people on the streets of the UK
Compassion in World Farming

Michelle has meditation CD's available:
www.purplebuddha.co.uk

Translation of Sanskrit words

Aklistah - non-painful

Asana - posture

Ashtanga: eight limbs of Yoga

Atma - true self

Chakra - wheel of energy

Chandra - moon

Citta: manas - mind, buddhi - intelligence, ahamkara - ego

Dharana - concentration

Dhyana - meditation

Dukha - sorrow, pain

Gunas - qualities of nature: tamas - lively, rajas - lively, sattva - light

Isvara - The Great Divine

Kaivalya - emancipation, freedom, liberation

Karma - fruits of past actions and lives - can be gifts or burdens

Khumbaka - breath retention

Kleshas: avidya - spiritual ignorance, asmita - ego, raga - desire, dvesa - hatred,   abhinivesah - fear.

Klista - painful

Kriya Yoga: discipline, self-study, connecting to The Great Divine

Mantra - sacred sound

Nidra - lucid dreaming

Niyama - attitude towards yourself

Pada - chapter

Perusha - the seer, the soul

Prana - energy, life force

Pranayama - breathing technique

Pratyahara - going inwards

Sadhana - practice

Sadhu - wondering spiritual seeker

Samadhi - beautiful blissful state

Samskaras - imprints from this life - your patterns that you are locked into

Samyana - integration of Dharana, Dhyana and Samadhi

Siddhis - psychic powers

Sthira - steadiness, alertness

Sukha - happiness, joy

Surya - sun

Sutra - thread

Svadhyaya - self-study

Tapas - self-discipline

Vairagya - non-attachment and renunciation

Vasanas - imprints from this life

Yama - code of conduct

Index

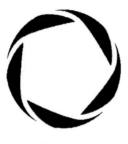

BOOKS

O is a symbol of the world, of oneness and unity. In different cultures it also means the "eye," symbolizing knowledge and insight. We aim to publish books that are accessible, constructive and that challenge accepted opinion, both that of academia and the "moral majority."

Our books are available in all good English language bookstores worldwide. If you don't see the book on the shelves ask the bookstore to order it for you, quoting the ISBN number and title. Alternatively you can order online (all major online retail sites carry our titles) or contact the distributor in the relevant country, listed on the copyright page.

See our website www.o-books.net for a full list of over 500 titles, growing by 100 a year.

And tune in to myspiritradio.com for our book review radio show, hosted by June-Elleni Laine, where you can listen to the authors discussing their books.

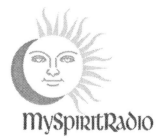

mySpiritRadio